The Life of a Seizure Patient

Darwin H. Hayes

If you have any questions or comments send them to
darwinhhayes@gmail.com All comments are appreciated

I would like to dedicate this book to a few special Doctors who contributed to this trying time in my life!

First: Dr. James Ferrendelli;
The neurologist who originally found my problem after watching me have a seizure at his office.

Second: Dr. John Miller;
The neurologist who took the place of Dr. Ferrendelli when he left and got me prepared for the process that was getting ready to take place.

Third: Dr. Dan Silbergeld;
The neuro-surgeon that done the surgery that changed my life.

Fourth: Dr. John Demorlis;
My family Dr. that has helped me in many ways too numerous to mention.

*   *   *

Darwin H. Hayes

Preface

The life of a seizure patient is something that a person cannot relate to unless they have been there to experience the effects that it has on a person. The picture on the front was chosen because it resembled the feelings that I experienced when I was told that there was no problem found when all the tests had been ran. I felt like I was on a road that nobody understood that could take me anywhere. The problem was that I wasn't sure if I was going somewhere that was better or worse.

The writings that I have here is a short version of some of the things that I went through that I wasn't sure what to expect but the only choice that I had was to hang on for the ride and find out.

If there are things that I have written that you feel can't be right all that I can say is that it is what I have experienced in my life. It is an established fact that every seizure case is different. I have no problem believing that because of what I have seen in the lives of the different seizure patients that I have talked to.

One thing that I must think about is the times that I went to doctors and neurologists and was told that I had no problem in my brain and still experienced the seizures that I was having. I went to doctors for almost twenty-five years before they found my problems and until that time I had people that thought that I wasn't really having the seizures that I was having.

When you read this, all that I ask is for you to think to yourself, what would I think if this was me. This is something that is hard enough to relate to when it is you and harder to understand when it is someone else. This is something that must be approached with an open mind or it is almost certain that you will end up lost and confused.

The Life of a Seizure Patient

When a person sees a newborn child, they can have many thoughts about how things are going to be for the life of their newborn bundle of joy. It's always nice to have a happy thought for what can happen with the life of a child that is the most precious thing in the world to you at this time of joy. The sad truth is that you never know what will happen in the life of this new person that has just been introduced to a world that is quite unknown.

When I was brought into this world I'm sure that it was no different than most births when the family and friends would gather and talk about the things that would and wouldn't happen. The sad truth seems to be that this life that we live does not come with a written guarantee saying that things will go perfect. That is something that is hard to accept when you look at the face and expressions of a newborn child.

My life went no different than most until I reached a point that would be a turning point for the rest of my life. Unlike many, that point was not 21 years old, or 18, or 16, or even 13 that point was when I was 9 months old.

I know, it's hard to imagine how a turning point could be reached in a child's life at nine months old but that is one thing that made my life quite different than most of the ones around me.

I was nine months old when I had my first Gran mal epileptic seizure. This was not taken lightly by anyone. The doctor told my parents that it was very possible that it could be something that would happen to me for the rest of my life.

My mother could not accept that to be the truth for her newborn child and it was something that would only happen this time never to happen again. This is something that I truly wish that she would have been right about but like I said before, this life has no written guarantees.

Life went on and things seemed normal for a child of my age and it was decided that it was not going to happen again. Little did anyone know that I was having seizures but I would hide from the world around me when I did.

I know that it is hard for anyone to imagine how you could go for six years and not know that something was wrong. When I would have a 'spell' I would go hide from everyone around me until it was over. I was the youngest of four children and it wasn't hard to disappear for a few minutes and not be noticed.

When I would feel a 'spell' I would go hide in my parent's bedroom closet because it was the quietest place that I could find and I would be away from all of the movement and noise that would bother me the most. I didn't know life to be any different so I presumed that everyone had these 'spells' and they had their own little hiding spots that they would go to until their 'spell' was over.

One day when I was six years old, my

mother came and opened the closet door while I was in there and she asked me why I was in their closet. The seizures that I had, made my speech go away until it would pass and when she asked me this question, no matter how hard I tried I couldn't answer her. She thought that I was playing when I first started this and I believe she got mad until she realized that I wasn't playing.

I can't imagine the thoughts that went through her mind when she noticed this, and the relief that she felt when she heard me speak to her after I went for a few minutes unable to speak. That was when the questions started.

She wanted to know why I didn't tell her that something was wrong. I can't say that I understand but I often wonder how she felt when I told her that I couldn't tell her. She gave me a look like she thought that I was trying to keep a secret from her and I had to explain that I couldn't tell her because I couldn't talk and by the time that I could talk there wasn't anything wrong with me I just had one of my 'spells'.

Of course, that just started a whole new

round of questions. I told her that I was alright and that was something that she did not believe. It's hard to explain something to a child that doesn't know anything different. When I told her that I thought that everyone had 'spells' she didn't understand how I could think that. She told me that everyone *didn't* have 'spells' and that made me wonder why I did.

Needless to say, taking me to the doctor was one of the first things on her mind at this point. From that time on she had questions to ask me that I didn't know the answers to and I think that just made her wonder that much more. She had to watch me closely from that point but to me there was nothing different than I had ever known life to be.

I went to see the doctor and had to answer all the questions again that I didn't know the answers to and I had to explain what I thought about the 'spells' that I was having. After I'd seen the family doctor he decided that I needed to see a specialist to determine what was causing the problems that I was having.

I lived in a town in rural Missouri that barely had four thousand people and to see a specialist I would have to travel over a hundred miles where there would be a doctor that was qualified to answer the questions that were being asked.

When we made the trip and I talked to the doctor he asked me to describe how I felt when I would have one of my 'spells'. That was something that I never could do simply because I couldn't think of anything that made me feel like I felt when I had a 'spell'. It was determined that I had epileptic seizures. The doctor thought that there was a good possibility that when I reached the age of around eighteen years old that I would outgrow them. He talked about it not being uncommon for children having seizures in the beginning of their life and outgrowing them when they reached the adolescent stage of their life.

The doctor put me on medicine that I would have to take every morning when I woke up, and every evening when I went to bed. I kept thinking that if I could take this medicine that I wouldn't have the 'spells' any more. That was something that I was disappointed to find out that I was wrong.

I had one sister that was nine years older than I was and I had two older brothers. One brother was eight years older and one was three and one half years older than me. My sister got married when I was eight years old and that was about the time that I started having gran mal seizures in my sleep. I would go to sleep in my bed and everything would be normal. I would wake up and would be in a hospital over one hundred miles away.

I think it was at that point that my sister thought that I was faking the seizures just to get attention. That was something that I wished that she was right about but she wasn't. When I started having the gran mal seizures the doctor put me in the hospital and ran some tests on me to see if they could find the source of the problems that I was having.

When I would have a gran mal seizure it was something that I would wake up like nothing had happened but anyone who was around me could clearly see that there was a problem. When the doctor would run the tests on me there wasn't any signs of any kind of abnormality to my brain waves on the

EEG that was ran. That made the doctor believe once again that I could possibly outgrow them when I got older. Not to mention made my sister believe that I was not really having seizures but just acting like it to get attention.

I reached the age of ten years old and started having some of the gran mal seizures at school, which started to be more of a problem for me when I would have them in class. Not only would I be disrupting the classroom but there was a strong possibility that I could hurt myself with all of the desks that surrounded me not to mention not being able to talk to the teacher to explain how I felt or ask permission to leave the class.

My parents had to explain to the entire staff at the school that I needed to leave the class as soon as I felt like I was going to have a seizure. When I first started leaving the classroom I would go to the bathroom because, like my parent's closet, it was the quietest room that I could find in the school.

After I did this for a while I started having gran mal seizures in the bathroom at school and the staff felt that it would be much safer if I would go to the office where I could be watched in case I did go into a gran mal seizure. I asked if I could go back to the bathroom because of all of the noise in the office from the typewriter and the people that would be in there talking as well as the phone ringing. All things considered they decided that it would be better if I was where I could be watched.

When I turned ten I was asleep one night when I went into another gran mal seizure and taken once again by ambulance to the hospital that was one hundred thirty miles from home. When I woke up that morning my mom was standing beside my bed and had a look on her face that I could not describe any better than to say that worried mother look. As soon as I opened my eyes she looked at me and with the same look on her face asked, "Do you know where you are at?"

I sat up in my bed and looked around the room that I was in and told her, "In the Springfield hospital." When I said that, there was a look of relief on her face that to this day, I can't describe. It was a look that was a mixture of happy to hear me talk and a look of relief to see that I was "going to be alright" The doctor decided to keep me in the hospital to have some extensive testing done on my brain to see if they could find my problem. After I was in the hospital for a few days and had testing done on my brain once again the same results came from the tests that we had seen before. There was no sign of any problems from the tests that had been run on my brain.

This point was like a dual edged sword, it was a good thing to still think that my problem was something that I would outgrow when I reached my upper teens but, it was also something that made everyone wonder why I was having my seizures.

By the time that I turned eleven I was beginning to work with my brother. We would mow grass to make money. This was questioned by many people. The doctor had said that I could be prone to having heat strokes so I needed to be very careful about staying in the sun for a long period of time. My parents were asked if I should really be out there in the sun working because it might cause my problems to get worse.

That was something that I never heard

a lot about until later when my dad told me about a few different times that question was brought up to him. The explanation that he had for the ones that would ask was simple. "He has to learn to deal with the problems that he has and make a life with what he has. If that is looked at as a disability it will be something that will stand between him and everything that he faces." He also told me later about a few different people that responded with an answer that really made them look at the things that I would do and watch me even closer. That response was "I never thought about that."

By the time that I was twelve years old I had a steady job that kept me busy most of the time. I found myself skipping doses of medicine and not having seizures and I'm not sure if I thought that the doctor was right and I had outgrown the seizures like he said that I would, or if I was just being stubborn enough to not want to take the medicine. I went for a time and found myself waking up in a hospital once again. This time I remember my mom and my dad looking at me when I regained consciousness and to see the looks on their faces reminded me of the times that I had seen that look before.

I later learned that the age of eleven or twelve was a typical age for many epileptics to do the very thing that I had done. That was deciding on their own that they no longer needed the medicine that they were taking. After I saw the results of this action I realized that the medicine was something that I was going to have to take and even though the doctor said that there was still a chance that I would outgrow this, something told me that the seizures was something that I was going to have to deal with, probably for the rest of my life.

I thought about what had been done by the doctor to try to find my problems with the tests that had been ran and by the tests not showing any problems it made me wonder if maybe my sister wasn't right, it was all in my imagination.

That was a thought that I didn't want to believe and I knew from the experiences that I had that there had to be more to it than what it seemed. There was a time that I was looking to see if the things that my mind was thinking could affect the seizures that I had.

I noticed that if I would keep myself busy between working on schoolwork and working on my job, it wouldn't allow my mind to wander on the thought of having seizures. That was something that I could not see as a cause for the seizures but I knew that something was causing me to have them.

When I was about fourteen, I was looking at things that would make for a life that could be dealt with by me. From everything that I had learned from the tests that had been ran and what the doctors had said I had to think about what was going on with my life and why they couldn't find my problem.

I had some thoughts about what I could do with my life, not only the things that could make a difference with the things that the doctors were doing to find my problems, but also the things that I could do, as well as not do, that might make a difference in my life.

This sounds like an odd thought, I will admit, for a teenager to be having. When a teenager thinks about how things are going on in their life it usually does not involve anything but the time that is right before them. This may not sound like something that the average person would think about, but I also had to consider that I was not exactly living what you would call an average life.

I think about the times when I would be at school and someone would ask me if I would like to go do something. I couldn't just change what plans that I had and go with a new one. I would have to consider if I had medicine with me that would be enough to last until I got home. I also had to figure that if we were doing something and I had a seizure would it be something that could be dealt with and go on, or would it be something that would spoil the whole time for everyone.

I also had to think about the things that I would do, that would affect me later in life. That was a time when boys usually start thinking about being with girls and started to get a different outlook about the life that lay ahead of them. When I had this thought, it was something that I wasn't sure what the best way to approach it would be. This may sound silly but I would like for you to think about it for just a minute.

When teenage boys get together to talk about what each other's actions are it is something that everyone can relate to because each one has similar feelings. My feelings were slightly different because I had to figure, what if I'm standing there and trying to think about what the best thing to do would be to meet this girl and in the middle of a conversation go into a seizure. That put a whole new light on the subject at hand. Something that I had to ask myself was, who else could relate to this point.

When a boy is meeting a girl, there are things that are done to try to impress that girl to leave an impression on her that can make her remember good things about him. I couldn't help but think in my mind about trying to figure out what to say to a girl and half way through a conversation start feeling like I was going to have a seizure.

I just thought that it might be easier to not even start to get the attention of the girls around me so I wouldn't have to deal with that issue that seemed to get the attention of more and more boys my age as time passed by.

I thought about what the doctor had said about me outgrowing the seizures but from everything that I saw they seemed to be getting worse. That seemed like a bad sign that needed to be thought about before rather than after it was too late to do something about it. I had to consider how I would feel if I would have a child that had the same problem that I had that nobody could explain. I decided that I could never forgive myself if that should happen.

I figured that if I didn't have a girlfriend then it would solve more than one problem that I was thinking about. It was easier to come up with a silly joke about it when I was asked why I didn't have a girlfriend than to try to explain something that the person that asked wouldn't understand anyway.

That was considered to be an odd way to look at things because it wouldn't accomplish anything, but I couldn't help myself but think that there was nothing being accomplished anyway. I had heard the same comment about me getting help for my problem so many times that it was something that I had a problem with.

I would enter into the emergency room at the hospital of a town that wasn't even a big enough facility to staff a neurologist. When I would enter in they would look at me and say about the same thing that I had heard before, so many times. The staff would say, "We will find out what is wrong we have the machines to run the tests necessary to find your problem."

I couldn't even count the number of times that I have seen the doctor walk back into my room and say with a surprised and confused tone to his voice. "We don't see anything wrong with you and it is something that you had better talk to your neurologist about."

I started running around with my brother when I was about this age because he had his driver's license and would run around with the people that were about his age. My mother didn't like for me to be away from her for very long at a time but it was something that she had started to accept at this time. She knew that I could have a seizure but it was something that she had realized that it wouldn't matter where I was at, it would have the same effect on me.

I have often wondered if that was something that she wondered about even when I would go traveling with my dad. He had a job that required a lot of driving to various places all over the country. That was something that I had done quite a lot of between traveling with him when he went somewhere for the company and when our family went on vacations I had been in a good portion of the United States.

By me being away from her as much as I had she had seen that it was something that I could do and I knew what to do if I felt a seizure starting. I would often wonder how she really felt about different things that I would do but it was something that I felt was not going to harm me and it was also good for her to see that I could handle a seizure if it should happen. I'm sure she was concerned but to be tied down to something is not always a good thing.

I had also noticed that there was very little that a person could do that would change the fact that I was having a seizure. Don't get me wrong if there was something that I was close to that I could hurt myself on they could try to keep me away from it as much as possible. That was something that I tried to prepare for when I felt a seizure coming on.

At this point in my life I could not imagine what a person went through when they see me in a seizure. I had never seen anyone have a seizure so I couldn't relate to the effects that one had on a person. I just knew how they made me feel. I know that this doesn't make any sense but when you stop and think about it you can see that it is hard to see things from another person's point of view. You also have to consider that I was unconscious when I had a Gran mal seizure.

When I turned fifteen I started going out with a girl that went to the same school that I did. This was a girl that I was around every day which was something that made it easier to get to know each other. It wasn't the first girlfriend that I had but it was the first one that I had since I had been thinking about the pros and cons of having a girlfriend as well as seizures.

I could see the advantages of having someone to be with, but I wondered about the things that might come later. I always heard different people say that you had to take life as it came but I couldn't help myself but think about the possibility of later in life having a child that would have to go through some of the same things that I had. My parents had checked into the history on both sides of the family and couldn't find anyone on either side that had seizures.

That was something that looked better to me as far as being genetic, but I couldn't help myself but think that everything has to start somewhere. When I thought about that I didn't feel any better about having a child that would go through the same type of life that I did. If it would have been something that was able to be found and explained I may not have felt so bad or unsure about it. With me going to a doctor for nine years now and still no answer it didn't make me see it any differently.

When this thought went through my mind I had to stop and ask myself again, are you just feeling sorry for yourself? It was something that I had asked myself so many times before that I was wondering about my own answer to the question that I ask. That made me think at least twice as hard about it before I answered and I continued to have the same answer.

When a person has to make a decision based on their own actions and life it makes a person understand why it is said that you can't be your own guinea pig. When you have a situation that no one else can relate to it makes this somewhat harder to come to a rational decision.

We stayed together for some time but after we had broken up I still had to ask myself these questions. At this point I decided to stay to myself as far as girls were concerned. There were times that I would think about being with a girl but I would have to think about what I had thought about before and what I had decided about my life.

I started drinking a little bit when I was about fifteen and I smoked some pot about the same time. This was something that wasn't untypical for a kid my age to try and I didn't see anything that made a difference with the seizures that I was having.

This was something that I watched to

see if there were any effects with smoking pot and having seizures. When I started smoking I began reading any literature that I could find about the effects marijuana had on epilepsy. I found that when the studies were done with marijuana there was a major contrast of different studies. That was something that made me pay closer attention. The more that I read about it I found out part of the reason for this.

When a study is done a good portion of the time it is financed by the government. I learned that when a study was done on marijuana, there were times that when the government would not get the answers that they wanted to hear the university would be denied the funds the next time they would apply for a grant. The Universities discovered that it wasn't profitable to do a study that had answers that the government didn't want to hear. When this was discovered there were many studies done that told them what they wanted to hear to assure future funding. That explained to me why there were different studies that were done on the subject that had different answers.

This made me do something that like I

said before is said to not be a good idea but I found that it was required if I wanted the true effects that marijuana had. I tried keeping my own records to get the results that marijuana had on me with my seizures. What I found showed me that the things that I had read about the varying studies that had been done were probably very true. It is a sad thought to me that the medical industry has more concern for their bank accounts than their patients. Enough said about that.

When I turned sixteen I was able to get my driver's license. I was able to get a job and have a steady paycheck and live the life of a typical teenager. It wasn't too long after this happened that my dad found out that the private school that I was going to had diplomas that were not accepted by many places to be legitimate. When he discovered this he told me that if I wanted to, I could go ahead and finish out my school there, or get my GED as soon as I quit school. I decided to get my GED and by doing this I had my diploma in my hand before my seventeenth birthday.

I had a job as well as went to school so when I quit school it was almost like I had every day off. It was very untypical for a person to have their diploma and be sixteen years old. This made it seem like I was older than I actually was and with me not ever going to high school and always running around with my older brother it made me run around with an older bunch of people than a typical person my age would. When I was seventeen the pediatrician that I had been going to since I was six decided that I wasn't going to outgrow the seizures and it was time to find me a doctor that could treat my seizures as an adult.

I had to agree that when I would go into the clinic to see the doctor it would make me feel like I was surrounded by a bunch of little kids. When I would look at the reality of this picture it made me realize that I used to be one of those kids. That was something that told me that I had truly outgrown the treatment of the doctor's care. When I would think about my situation in another respect, it would make me see things that presented themselves quite differently.

The thought of not outgrowing the seizures that I had been having, roughly from the time that I became a teenager, had presented itself as a reality now that would have to be dealt with for the rest of my life. The doctor had given up on the hopes of me reaching a point in my life that I would outgrow having the seizures. That was something that I was prepared for but the next thing was a little bit different. I had grown up with my parents taking care of everything that had to be done with the doctor and the medicine. Now I had reached the point that I would have to learn the responsibilities that were necessary to make the doctor appointments and get prescriptions filled.

This was something that I had a lot of help with because my parents wanted to make sure that I took care of all of the responsibilities that were required to receive the proper care that I would need to take care of the epilepsy that I had. I had been taking medicine for eleven years so that was nothing that I wasn't used to. Through this time of getting medicine I would go to the pharmacy with my parents and see the transactions take place that were required to keep my medicine supply. I also had seen what was required when something was changed or misunderstood by the pharmacy.

This might have been something that seemed odd for someone to stand back and see a young kid make a transaction at the pharmacy but it was something that I had been involved in since I was six years old. I knew that if there was a problem it was something that I would have to contact the doctor and let their office call the pharmacy to get the problem taken care of.

There weren't many times that I would have many problems because it had been seen many times in the past what would happen if I ran out of medicine. I had learned how important it was to keep my body medicine levels where they needed to be. I had tried to taper off the medications that I took and saw that I ended up in the hospital what I really wanted was to go through life and not have to take medication. I saw other people that would really like to take medications for any reason or for no reason. That was something that just showed me that a person is never happy with what life gives them so they try to do something that is different from their normal life to see what the change will be like.

It is so often that I have wondered if

they really know what they want and the more that I thought about it and the more that I looked at the people around me I saw that everyone was like that to a point. For all of the years that I had taken medicine and not wanting to and to see someone that wanted to take it for no reason was something that made me think about the subject with a quite different outlook.

When I thought about it and noticed the pattern that was followed I noticed that it didn't matter how I looked at things when someone looked at the life that they were living they were likely to wish that they had something different. That made me think more about the life that I was living and consider what it would be like if I had the life that I wished for. With all of the other people that I was watching, I saw that if I was to have the life that I wished for that I would find something else to make it something different than what I wanted out of life. This made me ask myself if it wasn't human nature to not be satisfied with what a person has.

When I looked at it from this point it made me feel that the seizures were something that made the goals that I wanted for the difference in my life much more reasonable than they might be if I didn't have seizures. It made me see that everyone had some sort of problem with the life that they lived, this just happened to be mine. This was my way of seeing that the seizures were something that could be dealt with in a way that would be much better than some other problems.

No matter how I looked at it, it was something that I would have to live with. I have seen people that would feel sorry for themselves or find reasons that they were not able to do something because of a disability. I tried to deal with a life that had been formed around the disability that I had. There were things that had to be considered from all angles and I tried to work around this instead of making it something that would stand in my way. There were times that I would have to totally avoid particular things but usually I just had to be careful not to overdo it when I done something.

As I got older I noticed that the seizures that I was having progressively got worse. Not only the intensity of the seizure but how frequent I had them. As I was growing up my dad had taught me many different things that he was able to do as well as the man that I worked for teaching me things that he was very good at. There was also different people that I knew that I had learned from that gave me a very wide range of different types of work that I was able to do.

After I worked at a factory for about a year I quit and spend the next year just doing odd jobs and running around acting like a teenager. During this time, I found myself drinking a lot more than I had been because there were many times that my friends would be having parties and I would be right there partying with them.

When I would drink alcohol, it was something that when combined with my medicine would give me a double effect. My medicine had drowsiness as a side effect and when mixed with alcohol it would intensify this effect. It would also have a bad effect on my medicine levels that my blood needed to maintain to have control over my seizures.

I found that marijuana was something that didn't have that effect on me or at least not to that extent. I found that I would rather smoke marijuana than drink alcohol but I would still drink. When I would go to a party I could drink beer but I noticed that after a few beers it would start to make me sick and I would have to slow down on the amount that I drank. If I could smoke a joint it would settle my stomach down to the point that I could drink some more beer.

I would find myself getting sleepy before the rest of the people would but I had to consider the down effect of the seizure medicine that I took that nobody else had to consider. When I thought about that I didn't think much about being the one that would leave early and not be able to drink any more when everyone else was going strong.

There was also another effect that I had to think about. When I did I figured that it was a good thing that I couldn't drink as long as my friends did. It stated on the prescription bottle not to drink alcohol but that was something that I didn't listen to I guess because it was something that I didn't want to hear.

I went for a period of time and found myself waking up after a seizure in an emergency room and when my drug levels were taken they were much lower than what they needed to be. I was supposed to maintain a blood level between ten and twenty. Since the alcohol killed this medicine it was impossible to maintain that level and drink alcohol. Considering this I found myself smoking more marijuana than drinking. I would still drink, just not as much.

I had been taking Dilantin since I was six years old the only difference was as I got older and my body developed and got larger it continued to take more and more medicine to control the seizures. It also had some side effects that I had for so long that I had got used to them. One of those side effects that I had was that it promotes body hair and facial hair growth. By the time I was fifteen I had a small beard and by the time I was eighteen it was developed enough that I found that I could go into some places and buy beer without being asked for an ID.

That was something that made it easier to buy beer and I was drinking more than I would have been otherwise. I was eighteen and old enough to get a wider range of jobs than I was before and my brother got me a job working with him so I could have a steady job and support myself. The only thing was that this job was five hundred miles away in a different state. This was the first time that I had been away from my parents and they weren't sure if I should do this but I went to see how it would work.

When I started on this job it was like any other job. There were things that I had to learn about the way that things were done and what the initial goal was that we had to accomplish. This was different than the job that I had before because I had worked in a factory and done the same job over and over again. This was something that we had a different type of job to do. As we would finish one part of the job we would move on to the next step that was different. The job that I had got was building grain elevators.

After I was there and got used to the job I realized that the drinking age in that state was eighteen. That meant that I could drink beer and go to certain bars legally. This was something that I thought was neat and I had to go to the bar just because I could.

I reached a point that I was going to the bar almost every night and was something that I looked forward to doing after we would eat. After I had made a habit of going to the bar I had a bad seizure and had to be taken to the hospital. When I got there my blood level was two.

When I saw the difference that going to the bar was making I had to stop drinking. This lasted for a while and then I decided that I could drink every once in a while. One night when I went to the bar I was driving home I decided that I needed to pull over and sleep it off and when I done this I failed to take the key out of the ignition and I was taken to jail. I was arrested for a DUI and had to do community service work as well as pay fines.

This was another incentive to stop drinking so I thought that I should slow down for a while to try to get caught up with everything that I had to pay for. I continued to smoke pot and it didn't have the effects on my medicine that the alcohol did. I started paying attention to this fact and tried to remember the things that alcohol was doing to me.

I would wake up in the morning to go to work and would sometimes have a hangover that I would have to deal with until mid morning when I would get to feeling better. I didn't have to do that if I just smoked pot. I would have a problem with my medicine maintaining an accurate level if I drank alcohol. Smoking pot didn't seem to affect my drug level. I could smoke pot and stay at home and not have to worry near so much about getting pulled over and getting into trouble.

There were things that I had to think about when I smoked pot but the overall affect that it had on me was much less than alcohol. I had to consider that pot wasn't legal but as long as I could keep it hidden and not run around making a fool out of myself I would be alright.

This went on for quite a while and I didn't have any problems. I had met people that I could get the pot from. I felt comfortable knowing that they were not affiliated with the law and I would be alright. The seizures seemed to decline as compared to when I was drinking alcohol. That was something that I couldn't help but notice.

I was five hundred miles from home so

I had found another place that I could call home even if it was for a temporary amount of time. I came back to Missouri to visit from time to time but it was a long time between visits when I would return.

After I had lived there for about nine months we finished the job that we had started and it was time to move on. My brother went to a different job that was about one hundred miles west of where we were working and I went to a totally different location. We were still working for the same company but were on totally different crews.

When I went to work for the other boss I was about one hundred fifty miles closer to home than I had been before. I went to work for this foreman and there were people there that also smoked pot that I met right away and they knew where the best place to get the marijuana was, so that was something that I didn't change. I would drink every once in a while, but nothing like I had done before.

It was shortly after I had came there that I had explained my seizures to my boss and he told me that he had talked to my former boss about that before I came there. Come to find out, he had worked for the boss that I worked for when he started working for this company. It was a boss that I had no problem getting familiar working with and he didn't seem to have a problem with me so we seemed to get along fine. I didn't notice a big change in my habits from this job site than what I'd had before.

I'd noticed that the world around me had accepted me for a person that could survive in a society that existed in an area and environment that was totally different than what it was when I lived with my parents. This was something that I had wondered about when I moved away from home and when I lived with my brother it was different but I still had my brother that could keep an eye on me and see that everything was done that I needed to do.

When I moved away from him it was more like I was going to have to take care of myself but the crew that I worked with had taken me in as family and watched over me to help me in case I needed it. This helped me to realize that there are people that will help you out if they see that you try to help yourself and try to help them out when they need it.

As I lived there for a little while I found different people that I got to know and tried to let them know what to do if I would have a seizure. It was to my surprise that there wasn't as much of a reaction that I expected from the people that I met. I met some that were familiar with other people that they knew that had seizures. This was something that I wasn't used to because there was a limited number of seizure patients that I knew from my home town. After I thought about this I realized that there were more seizure patients around me from my home town but it wasn't uncommon to try to stay away from people, more so than someone who had a normal approach to the lifestyle around them.

When a person starts meeting people from the world around them they find out that the people that you can meet comes from a much larger number of people than have been around. When you take the time to think about this you can notice that there is a lot more people that are similar to some of your characteristics than you first thought or realized.

This was a thought that I was surprised at but the more that I thought about it the more that I realized that I was better understood than I expected to be. I had been thinking that I was the only one that would understand what my seizures were like. When I found out that there were people that would truly understand some of the things about me that I thought was just me, it made me see that I was far from being the oddball that I thought that I was.

I'm not saying that they totally understood what to expect or how I felt but they seemed to have something to compare it to that made them understand better than I thought was possible. This made me relax a lot more about the possibilities of what would happen when I had a seizure. I would never know for sure until I had one and seen their reaction but just knowing that there was some experience in the past with a similar problem made me relax more about my surroundings.

This was something that made my life go more like a person would expect things to be. I was somewhat questionable about it until I seen that it was something they were used to being around. When I went to this new place it was 1983. I drove a 1969 chevelle and it was a car that didn't stand out too bad from the other models that were being driven at that time.

I decided to come back to my dad's house for a weekend and see some friends. I went to see a friend that I hadn't seen for a while. His dad was someone that I knew from when I had lived there before. He had a car that I thought was so neat that I had to try to buy it from him.

He had a 1964 Lincoln Continental that I thought that I had to have. I sat around and talked him into selling it to me and I bought it and left it setting at my dad's house. I went back to where I was living and took my chevelle and started looking around for a car that was like the one that I had just bought.

I went to a Ford dealership and asked the parts department if they had any parts for a 1964 Lincoln Continental. The man that I was talking to told me that they didn't have anything that old but I needed to talk to one of their salesmen. When he told me which man he was talking about I looked up and that man was already walking toward me. He walked up and asked me, "Did you say you had a '64 Continental?"

When I talked to him for a while I found out that he had the parts that I needed. Not only did he have parts for my car but he had a whole car like mine. We got to know each other and talked quite a bit and when I started having problems with my car I came back home and drove my Lincoln back.

It wasn't too long after that I moved back to Missouri and was living with my parents again and I was once again looking for a job. When I found a job it was at the charcoal factory once again.

It wasn't very long after I went to work there that I moved out of my parents' house and into a tent on their land. I lived in this tent from March to September. When I moved there I was working midnights so when I was there sleeping it wasn't too cold in the daytime but in September it was starting to cool down a little bit and I knew that winter was coming.

I built me a shack to live in and to some people it wasn't much but when I compared it to a tent, I thought that it was alright. When I built the house I was able to get electric which made things much handier. Before I got electric I just thought that people lived like that for centuries. When I could have electric it seemed like I was living a lot easier than I had been so I thought that I was doing alright. People still couldn't see how I could live without running water. I just figured that was something that I could get later.

From the time that I set up the tent it was seven years that I lived there without running water but I just lived about a quarter mile from my parents' house. I would carry jugs of water to my house to use for cleaning and drinking. I could take showers and do laundry at their house. This made it much easier than it sounded to most people who couldn't understand how I could live like that.

I was still having seizures but I figured that I had survived as many as I had it wasn't going to kill me. That was something that the ones who watched me have those seizures didn't hardly agree with.

This was a time when I was doing a lot of drinking and smoking a lot of marijuana and it seemed like the alcohol had more of a bad effect on me than the pot did. The main effect that the alcohol had was it would counteract my medicine. Once again, I got into the habit of drinking quite regularly. At this time, I was 19 years old and I continued to drink until I was about twenty two or so. I thought once again about the problems that I had when the alcohol would counteract the medicine that I was taking.

When I reached about twenty-two I thought once again that I was having many more side effects from that alcohol than I was from the marijuana. I started once again not drinking and smoking more marijuana because I knew from the past that I would have fewer side effects and it was much easier to deal with than to have the alcohol.

I could watch my seizures and see that I was beginning to have more than I had in the past and I wasn't surprised to hear some people say, "It's the pot that's making you have more seizures". After a few years, I found myself in trouble and I had to quit smoking the pot and guess what, I was still having more seizures. This was something that the people that were so dead set against the marijuana didn't want to talk about.

It was a few years later I went to University of Missouri/Columbia to their medical facility and it was a similar reaction to the ones that I had heard before. They put their top Epileptologist over my case. When he sat and read over my records he told me something that I had heard many times in the past. He told me that they could find my problem.

He put me in the hospital and ran all of the tests that could be ran to see what my problem was. I was on a recorder that recorded all of my brain waves except the time that they had me hooked up to the EEG monitors all day. One day while I was hooked up to their monitor the EEG Tec said that I started pulling the wires off of my head and she came out to stop me and got them put back on. When I came out of the seizure she looked at me and told me what had happened. When I was leaving that day going back to my room she looked at me and winked and told me, "I can't tell you this but (wink) I think they found something this time."

When she told me this I thought to

myself well after all of these years I'm finally going to find out what my problem is. I was released from the hospital and I returned to the doctor in about two weeks and was anxious to hear what they had found. I went in to see the doctor and he looked me squarely in the eye and told me something that to this day I can quote word for word. He said, "Mr. Hayes we have ran every test known to modern medicine on your brain and you do not have epilepsy."

I must have had the most disgusted look on my face that I could possibly have because he looked at me and said. "That should be the best news that you could possibly want to hear."

So, I looked at him and asked a very simple question. "What's wrong with me?"

He couldn't even look me in the eye and answered "We don't know."

I couldn't say anything about the Tech that had told me that she thought that they had found something because I didn't want to cause her any trouble. With the Dr. / patient confidentiality that could be something that could get her in big trouble and I didn't want to do that.

I noticed once again at this time that a person can look at someone else's life and have so many answers that in reality they don't truly understand. I saw that when you take the time to explain why you are doing some of the things that you are, they come back with that line that I had heard so many times. "Oh, I didn't realize that."

After I had heard that same line so many different times I found myself not even responding to many of the ones that would ridicule me for the things that I done. I found that it was something that they would feel better about thinking that they understood and had all of the answers and I would remain being the one that was too stupid to figure it out.

I knew more about my life and the surrounding circumstances than they even had a clue about and when I would take the time to explain to them what was truly happening with me they would always want to talk about something else that was much easier to deal with.

This may sound like I'm being inconsiderate of other people's feelings but I couldn't see that it was any different than them being that way with mine and it seems odd how many people want to overlook that little detail.

I continued to work at the charcoal factory until I was having enough seizures that I was missing so much work that I ended up being terminated for not being reliable. I still remember the day (or should I say night) that I was fired. I came home from work at seven A.M. and I laid down to go to sleep about an hour later. When I woke up I was coming out of a seizure and I looked at the clock beside my bed. That clock said that it was eleven forty-five P.M. and I was already late for work.

I had already been told that if I missed one more night of work I would be fired. I just rolled over and went back to sleep. I would not have been able to work and when I woke up it was six forty five A.M... It was just fifteen minutes before my shift ended. I called my boss and told him what had happened and he told me, "Darwin you are a good worker but you have missed too much work. I told you before that if you missed one more night that it would be the last one." I told him that I understood that and I couldn't help what happened and he explained that he understood that but he needed someone that he could count on to be there.

After I was fired from that job I started working for a friend of mine that had a mechanic shop in a different town. I would go and stay with him through the week and come back on weekends. After I had worked for him for a while I met a woman and got to staying late on the weekends and I ended up wrecking a car and moved back to my house. I went to work for my dad who owned a donut shop \ restaurant in town and he knew that I could cook and he needed a breakfast cook. I worked for him until the place burned. While I was working for my dad I ended up living with the woman that I was going out with.

This woman, who later became my wife, was with me one day when I had a seizure and she took me to the hospital to be treated. When she went, and got the EMT to come out to the car to take me inside he ran out to the car to get me and approached the car all gung ho to take care of the problem that she had told him about. When he came up to the car he swung the door open and saw me sitting in the car still in a convulsive state. She said he took a step back from the car and looked at her and told her, "We have dealt with this guy before and he gets combative. Why don't you sit here and watch him and if he gets any worse you come and get us?"

When I came out of this seizure she sat there for a while and after I had started to be able to talk a little bit she told me what had happened. After she told me this I decided that I had to pee. I walked up to the big plate glass window that had their receptionist sitting on the inside behind the glass. I walked up to this window and proceeded to "Take a leak". This lady sat inside watching me and sat there looking and covered her face and didn't know what to do. I just finished up and zipped my pants and got back into the car. Later, when my girlfriend told me what I had done, the more that I thought about this I started to remember doing it. After I thought about this for a while I remembered the reaction of the receptionist and I couldn't help but notice her every time I would go to the hospital, this lady would look at me and be embarrassed every time she saw me.

I worked for my dad in the restaurant until it burned and after that I went to work for my neighbor who ran a scrap yard. I had known the man that ran the place all of my life. His dad had lived there since I was born and he had moved away for a brief time and moved back when his dad died. I worked for him until I had a gran mal seizure there and he told me that he didn't have a problem with my work but if I was to have a seizure while I was around the scrap pile it could injure me bad or kill me and he couldn't take that chance.

It was at this time that I went to file for social security. I got statements from some of the places that I had worked which was the ones that had let me go because of the seizures. My dad had also written one about when I worked for him and said that if I wasn't his son and considering the problems that I was having he wouldn't have wanted to hire me for safety reasons.

I was approved for social security after eight or nine months and started receiving a monthly check. It was a while after I was approved for medicare I started going to Barnes Hospital in St. Louis. It was late 1994 I went to my first visit to Barnes to see a Neurologist. My girlfriend and I went back to the room and was waiting on the Dr. to come and see me. I went into a seizure and my girlfriend went to tell the nurse. She immediately went to get the Dr. who came in to watch me have the seizure. After he had watched me he done an exam and ordered a CT scan and an EEG. I had both tests ran on me countless times before and always got the same answer. When the results from these tests came back I went to see the Dr. and he told me something that I had never heard before. He told me that he had found the reason for my seizures.

When I heard him say this it was something that I had to sit and think about for a little while. This Dr. had run the same tests on me that other Drs. had ran in every facility that I had been in and each one had always told me that there was no problem that they could see. Now there was one that tells me after one round of tests that my problem has been found.

After I thought about this for a while I

thought about something, This Dr. had watched me have a seizure and like the tech in Columbia, he recognized abnormalities by knowing where to look to compare the readings of the test to my actions during the seizure.

When I went to the next appt. to see him he told me that he was leaving. When I heard him say this my first thoughts were that when I got another Dr. that he would tell me the same thing that I had heard from the rest of the Drs. that I had saw since I was six years old. I must say that was quite a depressing thought.

He assured me that what he had found would be seen by the Dr. that would be taking my case. The next appt. that I had I met this Dr. that would be my neurologist. When we talked about my case he told me something that I hadn't expected to hear. He told me that if everything turned out like it was looking there was a strong chance that after extensive testing was done that I might be a candidate for brain surgery. When he told me this it was something that I was skeptical about but I wanted to hear more about it. When he said that this was a very typical reaction that he heard from patients it made me feel a little bit better about how my feelings were.

It was at this time that I started looking into the possibilities of brain surgery and some of the things that it could help with and some of the things that could be bad about it. When everything was presented to me the good was heavily outweighing the bad. The thing that I wanted to see was someone that had done this before. When I started looking I noticed that it was something that was far from being a new thing.

I told my Dr. that I was interested in the surgery that he was talking about. He told me that there would have to be some extensive tests ran to make sure that I was a likely candidate. When this testing started, I spent a lot of time in St. Louis and that was something that I wasn't accustomed to. I was used to being in the country and now I was in the city about as much as I was in the country. I had a friend that lived-in St. Louis that I could stay with and that helped a lot. She was the one that had got me to go to Barnes and I was very skeptical because I had heard the same answer everywhere else so it was hard for me to see anything that would be different at Barnes. When I looked into all of the things that I could find it showed me that Barnes Hospital was a top of the line facility.

It was in the same time frame that Time Magazine came out with a rating on medical facilities in the world. It was to my surprise that Barnes was either number one or number two in neurology. That was something that made me feel much better about the surgery that I was getting ready for. When all of the test results came back it worked out that I was a candidate for the surgery that they were talking about. I told them that I wanted to do it and on September 13th, 1995 Neurosurgeon Dr. Dan Silbergeld removed a piece of my left temporal lobe. The test that they ran showed that there was a sclerosis of the tissue that was causing the seizures. When he went in to remove the sclerosis it was an area that was right next to the speech center in my brain. They woke me up after they were into my brain and marked the area that would affect my speech.

After they woke me up during the surgery I had to identify pictures and when he reached a point of my brain that affected the speech it was marked off to be the limits of the surgery. After the speech center was "mapped out" in my brain they put me back to sleep and removed the sclerosis. When I woke up from the surgery he told me that it was right up against the speech center but he was pretty sure that he had got it all.

There was something that happened that maybe I shouldn't say anything about (but me being the joker that I am) I can't pass up such an opportunity. When I went to meet the Neurosurgeon (keep in mind this is the guy that is going to work on my brain) for the first time there was quite an incident that I have talked about ever since.

We went in to talk about the surgery and what it would consist of and I took a friend of mine along that worked at Barnes and might help to give me moral support. Dr Silbergeld also had an intern (I presume that is what he was) in the room with him. With four of us in the room the surgeon started with a model brain taking it apart to show me the part of my brain that would be worked on. He showed me the area that would be removed from my brain and then I would be put back together.

After this had been shown to me he was still

describing to me what it would consist of when the surgery was done. He started to put the pieces of the brain back together and dropped a piece on the table. He picked up the piece that he dropped and carried on without missing a beat in the conversation.

He continued with putting the model back together and dropped another piece in the floor. He picked up the piece once again not missing a beat in the conversation. Still trying to put the model back together once again he dropped a piece on the table. When he done this he just scooted the pieces over in the corner on the table and still never missing a beat in the conversation.

At this point there was a time when all of the other three people in the room was about to bust out laughing. Considering the seriousness of the subject nobody did. This was some time before the surgery actually took place and nothing was ever said about this. After this time the surgeon and myself were always joking back and forth with each other. When I was on the operating table in the O. R. they were just getting ready to knock me out and when the anesthesiologist was putting the shot in the tube I looked up at Dr. Silbergeld and said, ("Dr. Silbergeld, Please don't drop my brain.") and I was out. I never heard anything about this and have often wondered if I was able to get it all out before I went unconscious. (I couldn't go without telling that part.)

After the surgery, I had a seizure while I was in the hospital. The doctor told me that it could be an effect that my body had from the surgery. I came home from the hospital about a week after the surgery and I was doing alright all things considered.

There was a lot of pain in my head where the surgery had been done and it seemed like my sense of hearing was doubled or tripled. When someone would whisper it sounded like they were yelling at me. After about five days at home I had a fever start again and the hospital was called and they said to get me there as soon as possible!

I went back to the hospital and was running a fever and had an enormous headache that I couldn't even begin to describe. I remember when we were going to the hospital there was road construction and I know that my dad was trying to make the ride as smooth as possible but I think he heard me cuss more on the trip to St. Louis than he had heard me cuss for all the rest of my life combined.

When we got there the staff didn't want to give me anything for pain until after they had taken a CT scan. My dad insisted that I be given something for pain because he could tell that I was in pain, bad pain. They went ahead and gave me a shot and took me to take the CT scan. I could sure tell why they wanted to wait on the pain shot after I started the CT scan. In the middle of the scan I started to vomit. This is something that after brain surgery is not a pleasant experience.

After the scan, there was nothing found that was wrong with where the surgery had been done. In fact, the whole time that I was there it was never determined why I had the fever that I had. I was given some very strong antibiotics until the fever broke and after I was sent home I continued to take some strong antibiotics.

After about two weeks the headache was almost gone but I would be reminded if I sat down too hard or anything that would cause a jar to my head. After the first month, it seemed odd to not have any seizures.

The surgeon had told me that there

would be a time that I would feel depressed after the surgery. My answer was, "Be depressed because I don't have seizures?" This was something that I couldn't imagine happening because I felt that it would be hard to be depressed about. When the time came, it was something that I had to tell myself, "Maybe they knew what they were talking about."

When I had gone for two months without seizures it was something that had been so long since I'd done that it was hard to remember. When I thought about this I couldn't think of when I'd done this before. I went for fifteen months without having a seizure and I had never done this before in my life, *EVER*.

When I had gone for about six or eight months I noticed that I couldn't remember things that I knew that I once had known. This is something that sounds odd but I couldn't explain the full feeling that I had. I started thinking of the time before the surgery that I had done some things on my own that I am sure helped with my ability to remember things from the past.

I sat and thought of everyone that I could think of that had ever taught me anything. I sat and thought of that person and the time that I had spent with them to try to move the things that they had taught me to different parts of my brain so it could be accessible after the piece of my left temporal lobe had been removed.

I started with my mom and my dad as well as brothers and sister and all of the school teachers that I had when I was in school. I went to all of the people that I had worked for to the ones that I had worked with that was able to teach me anything. This was a long list that a person never does realize until they have to think of it for any reason.

When I reached this point after the surgery I realized that there were more people that taught me things than I wanted to admit. This is something that made me think of things with a more open mind than the average person will think about. What I realized was that a person can learn something from any person that they meet.

This is something that is hard for a person to accept. A person naturally thinks that they are smarter than some people but you have to look back at the theory that no person knows everything. When you realize this, you can also see that just because you know more than somebody that doesn't mean that they don't know something that you don't.

When I thought about this I realized that there were many people that I hadn't thought of that had taught me something. This was something that bothered me to the point that I started thinking that in every situation that you are in there is always more than one way to get there.

I would bet that there will be some if not many that will disagree with this point but with what I have experienced I think that I have a pretty good argument. I tried to compare the structure of the brain to the structure of a house or anything that I had worked on before. I felt that there was more than one way to get inside my left temporal lobe than the way that I had always used before that had been blocked by the surgery.

I sat and searched for that access point and eventually I found it. That made it so I could remember things from before that I was having problems with. When this happened, I felt that I had figured something out that would do me some good to remember things and for that it did work pretty good.

There was something else that I hadn't thought about that could be an issue. That is the simple theory that where there is a way in, there is a way out. What I mean by that is that the information that I had stored that I couldn't find was now accessible to the rest of my brain to process and use for various things. But the thing that I hadn't thought about before was that it could also possibly open an access for the sclerosis to grow out and develop like it had done in the past and cause me to have the seizures once again.

After fifteen months, I had a seizure and it was something that I couldn't help myself but think that maybe I caused this to happen. Another thing that I noticed was that I could draw. This was something that I could never do in the past. I had always saw people that could draw and never could find in myself what it took to do this. I tried many times and never had any success.

I remember the nine-hour psych test that they gave me before the surgery there was a spot that I was told to draw anything that I could draw. I told her that I couldn't draw and she told me to draw whatever I could. What I drew was a crooked box with a pointed roof to be a house and two stick figures that were standing in front with a crooked sidewalk that went to this "house".

After the surgery, my wife had taken a picture of Dr. Miller, the doctor that got me lined up and ready for this surgery. I took that picture and drew a copy of it and took to my doctor. I told him that I realized that it was no Picaso drawing but told him to look at the drawing that I done before the surgery.

I also told him another thing that I could do that I never was able to do before was to write left handed. I had written poetry since I was about thirteen and at this time I was thirty-one. I noticed that the writing that I was doing after the surgery was a better form than it was before. I could see many things that this surgery had done to help me with doing different things.

After I started having the seizures again I was thinking of when I would have twenty-five in a month and it didn't seem too bad to have one every three or four months. When I would tell people that I had a seizure the first thing that they would say was, "I thought that you didn't have them anymore." I would have to tell them that when I would have one every three or four months that it was better than having twenty-five every month.

I must admit that when I had my first one I thought about the point that I was supposed to be fixed but when I would go for a while and not have another one it was much better than before. I noticed that every time that I would have a seizure that it would take me about three days to totally recover from the effects that the seizure had given me. I hadn't been able to go three days before the surgery without having another seizure.

As time passed I noticed that the amount of time that was between the seizures that I was having was getting shorter and shorter. This made me think of the way that the seizures had progressed before the surgery. When I had this thought, I was thinking of the worse. I thought that if they were to develop like they did before it would be something that would steadily get worse as time passed by.

When I had this surgery, the surgeon had told me that this was a onetime thing. If the first surgery didn't fix me, it couldn't be done again. As time passed by, I had an appointment at social security to be evaluated to see if I was still qualified to draw the disability that I had been receiving. It was decided that since I wasn't having as many seizures that I would no longer draw the social security.

I later found out from a different neurologist that I was seeing that the surgery could be done again but since I was no longer covered by medicare that I was no longer a likely candidate for the surgery. I've often wondered what the outcome would have been if I was still on the medicare. It didn't take long to figure out that if there wasn't some sort of insurance it was next to impossible to get the 'Proper medical treatment' that is always talked about when the subject of conversation is the type of treatment that is available.

The fact is that this treatment is available if you have insurance to cover the expense of the services that are rendered. Insurance is something that is impossible to get for a "pre-existing condition." Maybe I don't understand but I can't figure out how I could get any coverage since I've had seizures since I was nine months old. I've had insurance at the jobs that I've worked but as it is, nobody would want to hire me because of the liability factor that exists with me being a seizure patient. To get insurance coverage required to get this surgery done is something that is quite impossible from the things that I've seen.

When I think about this I often wonder if I'm going through another one of those self-pity things that you often hear people talking about. I would like to think that I'm not but I guess that is often said by the ones who are accused of this.

I've been told that there are more types of medicine that is available for seizure control. The fact is that when there is a new medicine introduced by a pharmaceutical company it is figured how many law suites this drug will have and the dollar amount that it will cost and how many patients will take this drug. This amount is then divided out among the patients that are taking this medicine for the first seven years.

After seven years the patent runs out that has been filed for by the original manufacturer. When this happens if there aren't as many law suits filed that was first thought, it will be manufactured by a generic company for a more inexpensive price. This is another example of you can have all of the top of the line treatments if you can afford them. Now considering this I find it hard to think that the pharmaceutical companies really do care for much of anything but the bottom line dollar figure that will go to their account.

When I thought about this and looked a little bit deeper all that I found pointed more in this direction than I first thought. I can't help myself but think that it has been arranged by those companies that the treatments that are available are the ones that can make money and some of the cheaper treatments that would work have not been presented to the medical industry for this very reason.

My doctor has tried a few of the medicines that I can afford and the ones that were tried have made very little difference. My medicine that I was taking was increased and it brought my seizures back down but I believe that the dose that I am taking is getting very close to a level that will do liver damage. This is one of the side effects of this medicine. Side effects are something that can affect different people in different ways. Some of these are minor and can go almost unnoticed. Others can be major and cause problems that can be irreversible by the time that they are noticed.

When you think about the overall picture that has been presented, it makes you wonder if the medical industry isn't using the patient (and charging them for it), as an experiment to see what the effects will be. If it kills them, oh well, they can call the next one to try something different. This sounds like a bad way of looking at the picture but if the actual truth was known, I think that it would be very close to what I was just saying.

If I have said anything that has made you mad about some of the subjects that I was speaking of let me tell you something that I say quite often. "It's not me; it's the truth that hurts." When the truth is presented in society as we know it there always seems to be a socially acceptable way of dealing with it. That way is to hire you a double-talking lawyer that can lie their way out of it and make it all sound good. The freedom of speech is only good in this country if you can afford to hire a lawyer to back you up in what is said.

I apologize for anything that has been said that has been offensive to you. It was something that I thought could make you understand the reason that I thought some of the things that I do. Like I said before I sometimes wonder if I'm just complaining more than I should.

After I had this surgery I noticed that some of the effects of the seizures that I had was quite different than it was before the surgery. I had reached the point before the surgery that when I felt the aura that I would feel before the seizure the seizure would develop in less than thirty seconds. After I had the surgery I would get this feeling about twenty minutes before the seizure. This would give me plenty of time to prepare for the seizure to happen. This sounds like something that may not make any sense but I found that if I could prepare for the seizure it would work out better than if I wasn't able to.

Sound has always bothered me when I would have a seizure. I'm one that always listens to the stereo. I have music playing at my house 24/7. I can turn the music down and go to the bedroom that I made to be soundproof. I built my house after living in the shack that I had built when I first moved to the place that I live. I added a room to the first place that I lived three different times and made a bigger place to accommodate the family that I had.

After I had been there for almost twenty years I built me a house that was built to make the way that I lived more comfortable than it had been. I had people that couldn't understand how I could live like I did but in the time that it took me to get the things together to build a house I found that most of them were still paying house payments or rent when I was done with mine.

I made my bedroom soundproof

because that was something that I had wanted ever since I was a kid. I have found myself when I feel a seizure coming on want to try to run away from the inevitable. This is something that sounds silly I understand but it is something that I can't help myself but feel. I noticed that there was some difference in the way that the seizures made me feel during and after the seizure. I found that during some of the seizures that I had, I was still aware of what was going on around me. It was a feeling of knowing what I wanted to say but not being able to say it.

This was something that made me think of the people that are in a coma and can't respond to the world around them. What is the possibility that they are laying there quite aware of the things that are happening and simply can't respond? This was something that I thought a lot about. I had to do a little more reading about the effects of the brain. I learned that there is more than one area of the brain that controls the speech.

One area does the thinking of the words that you want to say. This is something that makes the actions of the brain work much faster than the average person can comprehend. There is a second area that controls the muscles that makes this speech develop into words than can be heard and understood by those around you.

I can tell you from experience that it is very frustrating to know what you want to say and not be able to make the words so other people can understand. This is something that is very misunderstood by many people. It is similar to a person who has a major stuttering problem except much more intense and that is what makes me wonder and want to compare it to a person that is in a coma.

There have been many reports of people that come out of a coma and can tell the ones around them what has happened while they were in the coma. That makes me wonder how many coma patients truly do understand their surroundings. This is something that is disputed by many but I have to look at the experience that I've had that is similar and it truly makes me wonder about the reality of this thought.

By watching the effects that I was having before a seizure there are times that I can feel a seizure up to twenty-four hours before it develops. This sounds like a long warning but it is something that I had to pay attention to so I could be more aware of the effects of the seizure that was getting ready to happen. This is something that doesn't happen every time but it has been more consistent than I thought was possible. When I feel like this I try to not put myself in a situation that will be a hazardous place.

I do things that I've been told is dangerous but by me feeling the effects like I do I can prepare for this when it is getting ready to happen. Something that I enjoyed doing was swimming and fishing. I thought about the things that could happen if I were to have a seizure and decided that if I didn't do them at all I would be better off. After I had the surgery I could feel safer around water than before but I just never started doing the things that I had done before. I guess you can say force of habit or whatever you want to call it but that was another one of those things that it was easier to just avoid it than trying to explain it to somebody.

I work in a shop of my own working on cars and motorcycles and such. I've been told by the Doctor that some of the things that I do is dangerous but it is something that I can feel safe about because of the feelings that I get before a seizure. I have enough of a warning that I can step away from a situation before it develops.

I find myself having a feeling and stopping what I'm doing and this feeling will go away and I will continue. I have often asked myself if that was something that would have been a seizure if I hadn't had the surgery. I don't know that this is the case but I think that it is very possible. I think of the number of seizures that I had before and it is very possible that it would be this way.

There was a time about eight years after the brain surgery that I had what you could call a "bad year." In April, I had a motorcycle wreck that gave me a compound fracture to both bones in my lower left leg. It broke the ball of my ankle off, and I had an area in my shin bone that was missing about one and one half inches of bone. This inch and one half that was missing on one side of the bone angled down to nothing missing as it went across the bone.

The Doctor had to put a metal rod

inside my bone from my knee to my ankle. There were two screws put in my ankle to hold the ball in place for it to heal. I had two screws in the bottom of the rod and two screws in the top just below my knee. I had to give it time to fill in the inch and one half of missing bone. I went for three months smoking cigarettes and smoking pot and the bone wasn't filling in. I quit the cigarettes and smoked a little more pot than I had before. When I went back to the doctor he was amazed when he looked at the x-ray. The bone was filling in and the graft that he was talking about wouldn't be necessary.

I was glad to hear this because I had found out that the insurance that the lady had, was just going to pay for just over half of the cost of the surgery. I've been told that I could sue her and cover the rest of the bill but like many other things it was something that they didn't know "The rest of the story."

I had known this lady since I was eight years old and been friends with her this whole time. She was a person that didn't have any way to pay the bills that were charged for the surgery and hospital stay that was required to fix my leg. Everyone else thought they knew everything about the situation and tried to tell me what I needed to do, but when I explained to them what was going to happen they realized what I meant.

I was on crutches for six months waiting for my leg to heal. Just over five months after this happened my stepdaughter was found dead from a drug overdose and needless to say this was something that was quite a shock.

When I went back to the doctor he saw the bone had filled in and said that I could walk on a cane. I got some boots that had a top that came sixteen inches up on my leg to have the added support that I needed for my leg.

About three months later my wife and I separated. Like I said before this was a year that didn't seem like it could get much worse but I've always been told that no matter what happens, it can always be worse. There were many factors that took place but the way that things happened one right after the other it was something that just as the saying goes, added fuel to the fire.

During this year, there was some added stress that always causes the seizures to be more frequent. When I look back considering everything and how it happened the seizures could have been a lot worse.

After this time had passed it was like I had taken the time that it took to get used to the changes that took place. In some ways this change was easy, but in other ways it was something that was harder to get used to. My wife and I had been together for a total of fifteen years and when we had got together I was having several seizures every month and they were getting worse. When we broke up I was by myself without having the seizures so it was something that I can say that I'd never done before.

I'm not saying that I wanted to have the seizures but it was like my neurosurgeon had said about being depressed after the surgery because of the major change that was made. This was something that I didn't understand but when I saw the effects that it had I can say that it was quite different than I expected it to be.

When I got used to the life that I was

living it got easier because of all the reasons that we had split up was something that I wouldn't have to live with day by day. I started thinking of the time when I was younger and saw my seizures get worse as time went by. There were some places that I wanted to go to before I wasn't able to drive. I started traveling in the western part of the United States to see some things that I hadn't seen in my younger years.

There were many places that I had been but some of those places I was very young when I went and I wanted to see them again. There were some that I was curious about to see if they were like some of the stories that I had heard. I bought a car that needed the engine replaced and when I replaced it I drove it about two hundred fifty miles before I went to the Grand Canyon. When I went on this trip I had bought a camera about two days before I left. I started taking pictures so I could have them to remember my trip that I took.

When I returned from this trip I had something happen that I thought would never happen. I had written poems for almost thirty years and I had a few newspaper stories that were done about my writing. I had a reporter ask me if I thought that I would ever do any other type of writing and I told him "No this is the only style of writing that I'll ever do."

That was true for a long time after this story was written in the newspaper. When I returned from the Grand Canyon I had taken a picture of the canyon and I wrote a single verse of a poem to print on this picture. After I had written this, my style of writing totally changed. Everything that I wrote was written in a totally different style than the poems were. I looked at a picture of a rock that I had taken before I got to the canyon and I said, "This looks like a castle, The Castle of Thiendra."

When I said this, I questioned myself about where this name came from and never figured it out. It was about three and one half months later that I started writing what has turned into a book that I got a contract for through a publishing company.

I worked on writing this story for almost a year and one half and turned it in to the publishing company and was presented a contract for it. I have written several papers that have been a totally different style than the poems that I was used to writing. Since I started on this story I haven't written another poem. I could never figure out what made me change I just knew that I did.

After I started writing the story, I took a few more trips looking for the inspiration that I needed to finish this story. By the time that I had finished the manuscript that I presented to the publisher I had been in every state west of the Mississippi River except three and some of them more than once. I had also been in seven states east of the Mississippi River.

I've been asked why I traveled so much while I was writing this story but I must say that it was a way for me to find the inspiration necessary to finish the story. There were many different landscapes in the states that I was in and to see them and compare them to some of the others, it made the contrast that it took to relate to the story and how to make everything come together and fit in with each time that it would change.

When I had completed these trips, I had been in all of the forty-eight states in the continental United States. This was something that I had thought a lot about in the years that it took to cover them all. There are many places that I haven't been but I have been in three provinces of Canada as well as the forty-eight states. Now I want to go to Alaska and Hawaii to say that I have been in all fifty states.

I can't say that I never have seizures now but there is quite a difference in how they are. There was one seizure that I had when I was alone that is one that is "quite different than other ones. The woman that I was with had talked to me and said that she was going to come to my house and see me and I told her that I would be at home. After we had talked on the phone, there was some time had passed and I felt a seizure coming on and I went into my bedroom and laid down.

When she came to the house she didn't see me and came into the house and I wasn't there. She looked outside and saw my dog looking out into the woods. When she looked out toward the area that the dog was looking she saw me. I was out in the woods with no clothes on at all wandering around. She went out to where I was and asked me what I was doing and realized that I was having a seizure. She walked me back to the house and got into the bedroom and laid me down until the seizure was over.

When I regained consciousness, she was explaining to me how she had found me and told me what had happened and I didn't remember anything that she was describing I had seen times that I couldn't remember anything about the time I was in the seizure and I had seen times that I could remember the seizure and the things that happened around me.

One time I was driving home from the pharmacy and had just picked up my medicine and felt the seizure coming on. I pulled off of the highway and after I had sat there for some time I went into the seizure. When I reached a point that I was able to remember the things that were going on around me I saw a deputy sheriff that was watching me and keeping me off of the road. When an ambulance arrived there were two EMTs that were in it and when they started to load me into the ambulance I tried to tell them that I didn't want to go to the hospital.

One of them had seen the medicine that I had just got from the pharmacy and looked at the price tag that was attached to the unopened bag. When he saw how much this medicine had cost he made the statement, "He must be selling these because nobody pays this much for drugs and doesn't sell them."

When I heard him say this I didn't want to be loaded into the ambulance and I still couldn't talk. I stood up beside my pickup and put my arm inside the door to hang on to hold myself up when I wouldn't let go and they couldn't get me loaded into the ambulance they physically pulled me from the truck and put handcuffs on me and forcefully loaded me in the ambulance. I knew that there was nothing that the hospital would do for me except run up the bill for doing nothing that would help.

I will say once again that I do not mean to try to make it sound like I know more about everything than the hospital workers do, but I do know how these same results have turned out in the past. When everything was done, the doctor knew nothing more than he had known before except that he couldn't do anything that would make a difference and had almost a thousand dollars' worth of medical bills.

Just before I was released I heard the same EMT still talking about not knowing what the pills were for that I had just picked up at the pharmacy. His partner came up behind him and said in a tone of voice that told me that he had looked them up in the same book that was accessible to both of them, "They are for seizures". This was something that told me that the man who was driving the ambulance was one that would look into things before he jumped to conclusions. This made me feel much better about him but his partner is one that needs to take the time to learn about the things that are a part of his job.

I'm glad to say that with the adjustments that have been made with my medicine there has been a decrease in the number of seizures that I am having instead of the increase that I was so afraid of when I started traveling this last time. I'm hoping to see this pattern continue so I will never have to see the time when I have as many seizures as I have experienced in the past but I guess the only thing that I can do to find out is like I said in the preface, "Hang on for the ride and see where it takes me"

I would like to thank you for taking the time to read the things that I have written. I truly hope that it has made you understand some things that you have been questionable about in the past. When I think that a person can better understand a situation by reading what I have written, it gives me a sense of accomplishment that I can think that maybe all of the things that I have experienced in my life can be useful to understand a disease that has been very much misunderstood in the past.

Darwin H. Hayes

About the Author

Darwin H. Hayes was born in Missouri and lived there all his life except for one year. He started writing when he was 13 years old and wrote poetry for almost thirty years. Five of his poems were made into songs and recorded on albums. After he had brain surgery that was done for the seizures that he had from birth, there was a change in his way of seeing things to write about.

He was inspired to write in a different style than had been known to him before that time. The result of that inspiration was a story that would be made into a book to be presented to the public. This book was the beginning of his writing style that has become a habit for him to follow. It has been said that he has a twist in his descriptive ways of writing and that is something that he did not change when he started writing in a different style.

www.ingramcontent.com/pod-product-compliance
Lightning Source LLC
Chambersburg PA
CBHW062052280526
45788CB00003B/1207